PHYSICK

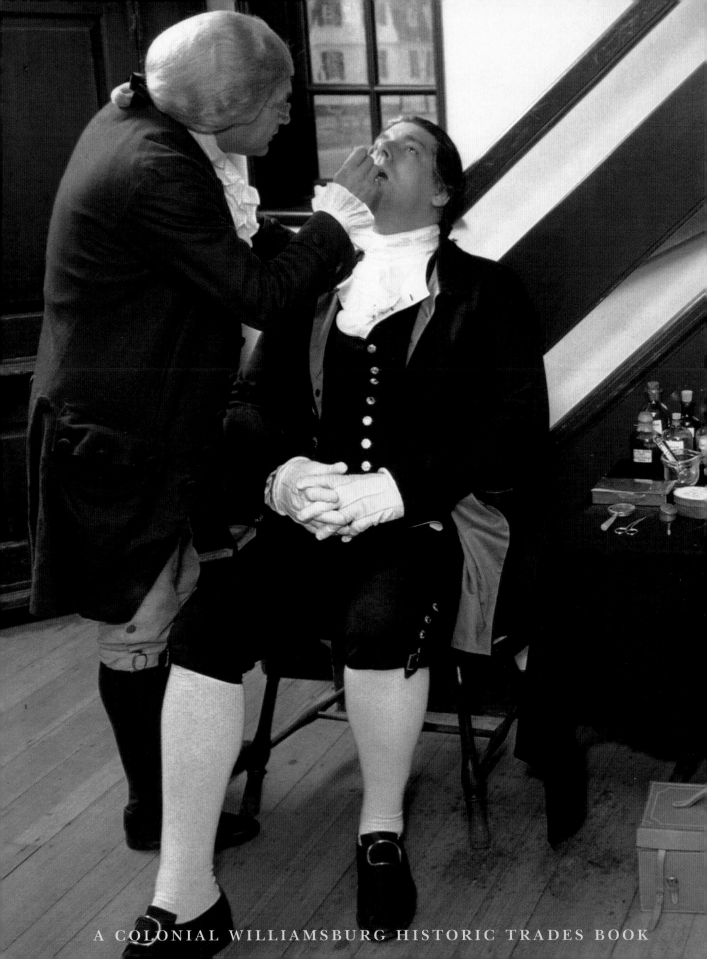

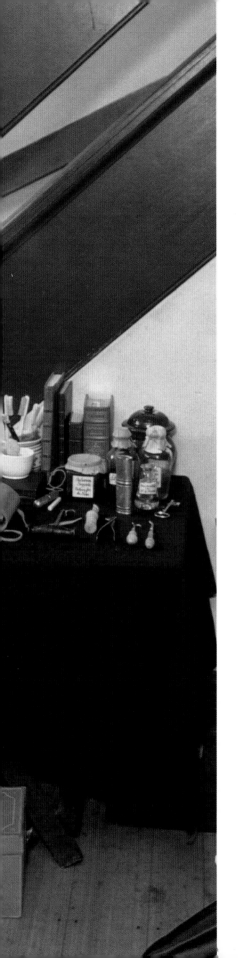

PHYSICK

The Professional Practice of Medicine in Williamsburg, Virginia, 1740–1775

TEXT BY

Sharon Cotner
Kris Dippre
Robin Kipps
and Susan Pryor

PHOTOGRAPHY BY

David M. Doody

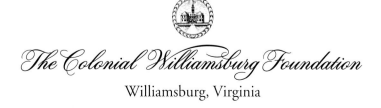

The Colonial Williamsburg Foundation

Williamsburg, Virginia

Library of Congress Cataloging-in-Publication Data

Physick : the professional practice of medicine in Williamsburg, Virginia, 1740–1775 / by Sharon Cotner . . . [et al.].

    p. ; cm.

Includes bibliographical references.

 ISBN 0-87935-219-1 (alk. paper)

 1. Medicine–Virginia–Williamsburg–History–Colonial period, ca. 1600–1775. 2. Pharmacy–Virginia–Williamsburg–History–Colonial period, ca. 1600–1775.

 [DNLM: 1. History of Medicine, 18th Cent.–Virginia. WZ 70 AW2 P578 2002] I. Cotner, Sharon. II. Colonial Williamsburg Foundation.

 R346.W54 P48 2002

 610'.9755'425209033–dc21

2002154056

Designed by Helen M. Olds

Printed and bound in China

Acknowledgments

The Colonial Williamsburg Foundation and its staff at the Pasteur and Galt Apothecary gratefully acknowledge the support of the Merck Company Foundation and the Ambrose and Ida Fredrickson Foundation whose financial contributions made the research and publication of this book possible. Individuals who generously contributed include Mr. and Mrs. Richard C. Brand, Jr., Dr. and Mrs. Ira E. Lew, and Mr. Trevor Woodward. Thank you for being partners with us in exploring and sharing the history of medicine. A special thank you from the authors is extended to the employees and interns who assisted us in completing this endeavor. We would also like to thank our families and co-workers for their interest in and encouragement of this project.

Note to the Reader

The focus of this work is the professional practice of medicine in Williamsburg between 1740–1775. Williamsburg's medical profession was dominated by men trained in the European tradition of medicine. Some of the featured topics include medical theory, education, treatments, surgery, and brief biographical sketches of several local practitioners. The lay practice of medicine including domestic and folk medicine has been omitted due to space constraints.

The four authors are specialists in eighteenth-century medical history. We have worked together at the Pasteur and Galt Apothecary Shop for the Colonial Williamsburg Foundation since 1984. Each has focused her study on a different aspect of medical history. As a result, each major topic has been written by a different author using the clinical practice of medicine in Williamsburg as a unifying theme. The goal of this book is to present the material in an understandable and interesting manner to those who have had little time to read about medical history and to share the authors' enthusiasm for studying Williamsburg's history.

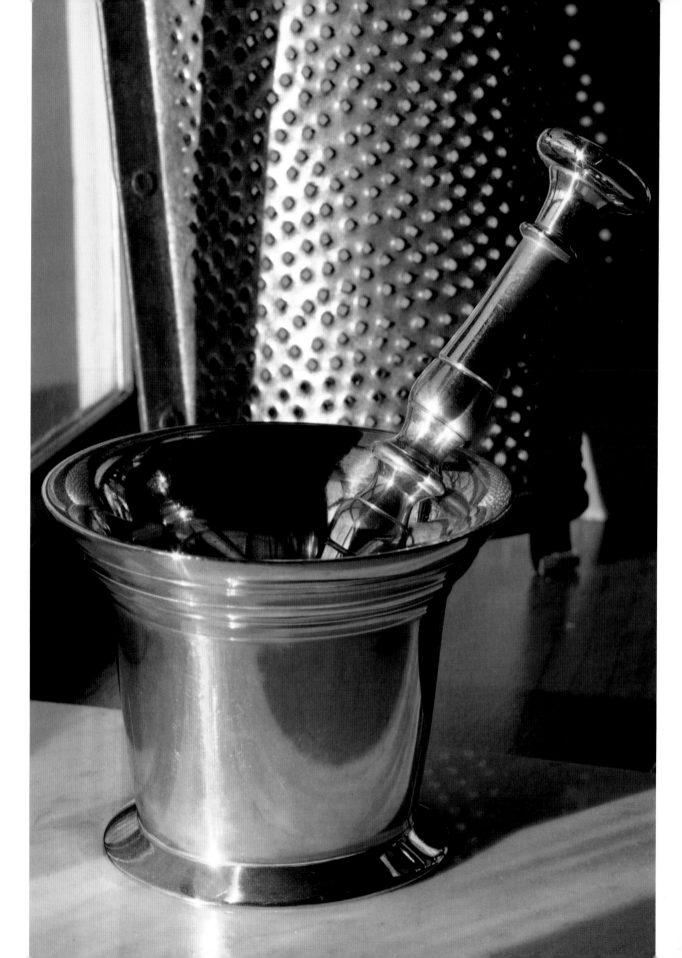

ON SEPTEMBER 23, 1770, in Williamsburg, Virginia's royal governor, Norborne Berkeley, Baron de Botetourt, "was taken with a Slight fever . . . which he got the better of, it returned in a week after, he . . . did not consider himself in a dangerous Situation till the Friday before he died . . . [when] he had three fits in which he was Greatly Convulsed." So wrote James Parker to his friend Charles Steuart in London in December 1770.[1] Dr. John de Sequeyra and local apothecary Dr. William Pasteur attended to the governor and declared his illness to be of two ailments, a bilious fever and St. Anthony's Fire, or erysipelas, a bacterial infection. Dr. de Sequeyra further described Lord Botetourt's case: His "Blood being in a bad condition, it turned of the Malignant kind, having large Spots of a purple Colour upon his Breast & part of his Back."[2] He told the patient that there was no hope of recovery. "On Sunday being given over by the Doct. the treasurer [Robert Carter Nicholas] and some others who were there gave him a Dose of Jameses powders, which Mr. Nicholas . . . thought relieved him a little, he Died about one o'clock on Monday morning, 15th Oct."[3]

Lord Botetourt was able financially to afford professional medical attention during his illnesses and requested two of Williamsburg's leading medical professionals. Most of the community's affluent citizens followed the same course for themselves and their families and slaves. They paid well for such a luxury. In November 1792, Miles King, Esq., paid Dr. John Minson Galt £27.12.6 for thirteen days' attendance for smallpox.[4]

Mortars and pestles came in different sizes and were made from a variety of materials.

The gentry were not the only ones who sought the services of professional doctors. Those of more modest means also favored professional treatment over domestic practice. Dr. Galt and Dr. Thomas Wharton identified many patients by profession in their account books: John Jones, carpenter; John Carter, carter; Mr. Morris, player; and John Davis, sailor. Some widows or single women such as Mrs. Mary Brown and Miss Nancy Wray maintained their own accounts.[5] Slaves appeared frequently as patients in Dr. Galt's daybooks. Treatments were charged to their masters' accounts.

Itinerant practitioners who often charged lower rates but may have possessed dubious credentials sometimes came to town. Dr. Graham, an oculist and aurist, arrived in Williamsburg in the spring of 1773. His advertisements in the *Virginia Gazette* targeted "those persons whose Circumstances or Situation have precluded them from the Benefit of applying for Assistance at Philadelphia . . . in all disorders of the Eye and its Appendages, and in every Species of Deafness, Hardness of Hearing, Ulcerations, Noise in the Ears, etc."[6] According to testimonials, he restored sight to Miss Peggy Hay after a lengthy blindness as a result of a *gutta serena* (blindness with no apparent cause).[7] Others blinded by cataracts also had their sight restored as the result of his ministrations. During his brief stay in Williamsburg, Dr. Graham was so overwhelmed with patients from all over the colony that he placed a note of apology in the *Virginia Gazette* to those he was unable to treat.[8]

Others suffered from illnesses so cruel and unsparing that they desperately sought treatment from any source. On June 6, 1777, William Hansbrough of Amherst County advertised in the *Gazette* beseeching *anyone's* assistance in the successful treatment of his cancer.[9]

Although medical professionals in Williamsburg throughout the eighteenth century had been educated in various ways, the fewer than two thousand residents of the town were unable to support much specialization. This may explain why itinerants with specialties—such as Dr. Graham—were popular.

Credit was extended to both men and women. The debt was paid with currency that the doctor could use to buy supplies and pay creditors in England.

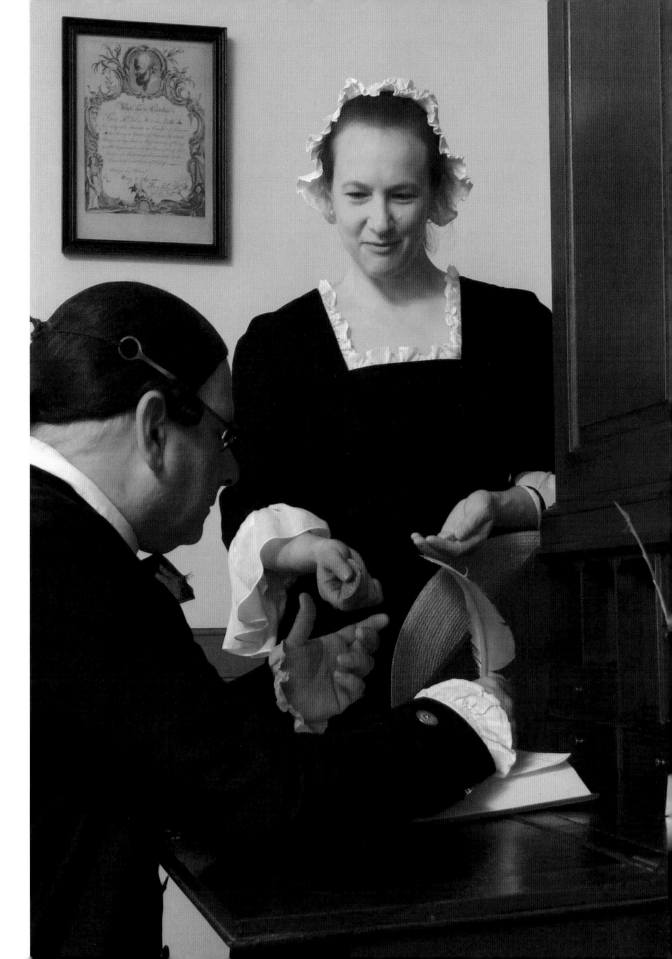

Training by Apprenticeship

In Great Britain, practitioners specialized as physicians, apothecaries, druggists, surgeons, tooth drawers, midwives, and others. Traditionally, a physician was concerned with internal disease. He was university trained, although he may have completed an apprenticeship as well. An apothecary was almost always apprentice trained. He not only compounded and dispensed medicine but prescribed treatment. Druggists made and sold medicines but did not engage in active practice. Surgeons limited their work to manual labor, performing treatment for wounds, fractures, tooth extractions, operations, and the like.

In Williamsburg, the medical professional usually combined these specialties into one as an apothecary-surgeon dispensing medicine, giving advice, and performing surgery. No matter what his education, he was most commonly referred to as "doctor." While there were physicians, apothecaries, apothecary-surgeons, and even a druggist for a short time, there were no professional surgeons in the town.

Although the demands of the profession in America would seem to have required medical training of some sort, standards of quality established by guilds, licenses, or guidelines did not exist in Virginia or elsewhere in the colonies. In fact, there was no legal requirement that practitioners receive medical education at all.

Virginia was not entirely devoid of educational opportunities in medicine, however. Apprenticeships were common and usually contracted for five to seven years, although the term was not absolute. The vast majority of Williamsburg's doctors trained by apprenticeship and, in turn, trained others. Doctors John Minson Galt, William Pasteur, Robert Nicolson, and Andrew Anderson all apprenticed. Frederick Bryan's 1778 apprenticeship indenture with Dr. Galt clearly illustrates the restrictions and duties imposed on apprentices:

This Indenture Witnesseth that Frederick Bryan an Infant about the age of eighteen years Orphan of Frederick Bryan late of the County of York decd by and with the Consent and approbation of the Justices of the Court of the said County Hath put himself and by these presents Doth put himself apprentice to John Minson Galt *of the City of Williamsburgh* Apothecary *to learn his Art and Mystery and after the manner of an Apprentice to serve the said John Minson Galt from*

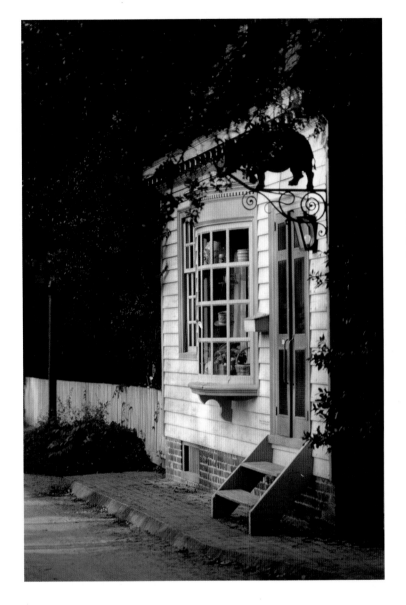

Dr. George Pitt's office was located at the Sign of the Rhinoceros on Colonial Street. Today, it is a private residence.

the day of the date hereof for and during and unto the full end and term of four Years during att which term the said Apprentice his said Master faithfully shall serve his Secrets keep his lawful commands at all times shall readily obey He shall do no damage to his said Master nor see it to be done by others without giving Notice thereof to his said Master. He shall not commit fornication nor contract Matrimony within the said term; At Cards Dice or any other unlawful game he shall not play whereby his said Master may have damage With his own Goods or the Goods of others without Licence from his Master he shall not buy or sell He shall not absent himself Day or Night from his said Masters Service nor haunt Ordinarys Taverns or Playhouses but in all things behave himself as a faithful apprentice ought to do during the said Term.

And the said Master shall do the utmost of his endeavours to teach and instruct or cause to be taught and instructed the said Apprentice in the Art and Mystery of an Apothecary and find and provide for him good and sufficient Meat Drink and Lodging fitting for an apprentice during the said term and for the true performance of all and singular the Covenants and Agrements aforesaid the Parties bind themselves each unto the other firmly by these presents.

In Witness thereof the said Parties have hereunto set their hands and affixed their Seals this sixteenth day of November [1778.][10]

Although Virginia offered no formal training in medicine, several Williamsburg doctors complemented their apprenticeships with hospital or university training abroad. Both William Pasteur, who received financial assistance from his former master, George Gilmer,[11] and John Minson Galt attended St. Thomas's Hospital in London for at least a year. Andrew Anderson augmented his apprenticeship with James Carter by studying in hospitals and doing course work in England. George Gilmer, Sr., received medical education at Edinburgh and sent his son there as well. Williamsburg doctors also earned medical degrees from European universities. Dr. John de Sequeyra received his degree from the University of Leiden in Holland in 1739, and Dr. James McClurg's degree was from the University of Edinburgh in 1770.

The organization of Edinburgh's medical school provided the basis for America's first two medical schools. The first was established in 1765 at the College of Philadelphia, which later became the University of Pennsylvania. Admission to the school required degree candidates to have a bachelor's degree or its equivalent and to prove proficiency in pharmacy by having served at least a three-year apprenticeship. The bachelor's degree required at least one course in anatomy, materia medica, chemistry, and the theory and practice of medicine, as well as clinical lectures. It also required one year's attendance at the Pennsylvania Hospital. A doctor's degree was awarded after completing three years of professional experience and the required composition and public defense of a thesis in Latin. America's second medical school opened in 1767 at King's College in New York and offered very much the same curriculum. After the Revolution, the school was renamed Columbia University.

Through Thomas Jefferson's influence on the board of visitors in 1779, the College of William and Mary created a chair in anatomy and medicine to which Dr. James McClurg was appointed. Four years later, in 1783, the chair was discontinued. Dr. McClurg resigned from the faculty for unknown reasons and moved to Richmond. Just how much teaching, if any, he did is also unknown.

Standards of Quality

In spite of numerous and varied methods of training available to doctors in the colonies, there were no standards of quality, and the enforcement of the few regulations that did exist was left up to each individual colony. The earliest colonial regulations imposed on medicine in Virginia concerned overcharging for services, and by 1667, the establishment, when necessary, of quarantine facilities for smallpox patients. Occasionally, legislation concerning the criminal neglect of patients and ethics was enacted, yet there was no regulation of the practitioners themselves. One such effort to control overcharging in Virginia was the enactment in 1736 of a fee schedule that was in effect for at least two years. This schedule set some fees according to the practitioner's education level. Additional bills for regulating fees introduced in 1748, 1761, and 1762 were defeated.

Virginia took an active—although futile—role in the effort to legislate doctors. William Langhorne, a burgess from Warwick County from 1772 to 1774, addressed the General Assembly, asking "Would it be wise in the Virginia Legislature to require examination and license of persons proposing to practice medicine?" Langhorne argued:

Before a man should be permitted to undertake the highly important duties of a physician he should be perfectly acquainted with the curious structure and œconomy of the human system; the history of the various diseases, their remote and subtle symptoms, and the mode of ascertaining and combatting them. . . . If it is necessary that every one intending to practice medicine should be thus qualified, is it not necessary that their fitness should be certified to the public by persons capable of judging officially . . . in order that the ignorant part of the community may have some assurance that the man to whom they are about to submit their constitutions and their lives is

I

Whereas the practice of phisic in this colony, is most commonly taken up and followed, by surgeons, apothecaries, or such as have only served apprenticeships to those trades, who often prove very unskilful in the art of a phisician; and yet do demand excessive fees, and exact unreasonable prices for the medicines which they administer, and do too often, for the sake of making up long and expensive bills, load their patients with greater quantities thereof, than are necessary or useful, concealing all their compositions, as well to prevent the discovery of their practice, as of the true value of what they administer: which is become a grievance, dangerous and intolerable, as well to the poorer sort of people, as others, & doth require the most effectual remedy that the nature of the thing will admit:

II

Be it therefore enacted, by the Lieutenant-Governor, Council, and Burgesses, of this present General Assembly, and it is hereby enacted, by the authority of the same, That from and after the passing of this act, no practicer in phisic, in any action or suit whatsoever, hereafter to be commenced in any court of record in this colony, shall recover, for visiting any sick person, more than the rates hereafter mentioned: that is to say,

Surgeons and apothecaries, who have served
an apprenticeship to those trades, shall be allowed,

	£	s	d
For every visit, and prescription, in town, or within five miles,	00	5	00
For every mile, above five, and under ten,	00	1	00
For a visit, of ten miles,	00	10	00
And for every mile, above ten,	00	00	06

With an allowance for all ferriages in their journeys.

(Above and opposite) **Enacted in 1736 by the Virginia House of Burgesses, this act, which set the practitioner's fees according to his educational level, remained in effect for at least two years.**

	£	s	d
To Surgeons, For a simple fracture, and the cure thereof	02	00	00
For a compound fracture, and the cure thereof,	04	00	00
But those persons who have studied phisic in any university, and taken any degree therein, shall be allowed,			
For every visit, and prescription, in any town, or within five miles,	00	10	00
If above five miles, for every mile more, under ten,	00	1	00
For a visit, if not above ten miles	1	00	00
And, for every mile, above ten,	00	1	00
With an allowance of ferriages, as before.			

III

And to the end the true value of the medicines administred by any practicer in phisic, may be better known, and judged of, *Be it further enacted, by the authority aforesaid,* That whenever any pills, bolus, portion, draught, electuary, decoction, or any medicines, in any form whatsoever, shall be administred to any sick person, the person administring the same shall, at the same time, deliver in his bill, expressing every particular thing made up therein; or if the medicine administred, be a simple, or compound, directed in the *dispensatories*, the true name thereof shall be expressed in the same bill, together with the quantities and prices, in both cases. And in failure thereof, such practicer, or any apothecary, making up the prescription of another, shall be nonsuited, in any action or suit hereafter commenced, which shall be grounded upon such bill or bills: Nor shall any book, or account, of any practicer in phisic, or any apothecary, be permitted to be given in evidence, before a court; unless the articles therein contained, be charged according to the directions of this act.

IV

And be it further enacted, by the authority aforesaid, That this act shall continue and be in force, for and during two years, next after the passing thereof, and from thence to the end of the next session of assembly.

competent to the task which he undertakes? . . . I appeal to your good sense to determine whether or not it is a subject worthy the attention of our legislature and if it would not be wise in them to secure their fellow citizens against fraud and imposition by inhibiting all persons from attempting to practice medicine without undergoing a regular examination and presenting a certificate of their competency.[12]

Unfortunately, Langhorne's words precipitated no change in the opinions or actions of the burgesses. Around 1870, America finally began to enforce nationwide standards of medical education and grant licenses to practice.

Medical Practices

Medical practices in colonial Williamsburg were rooted in European tradition. The predominant theory governing the practices in the eighteenth century resulted from combining traditional philosophies and new scientific discoveries. The Scientific Revolution, which began in the seventeenth century, did not immediately have an impact on the practice of medicine. However, older theories were undergoing some fundamental changes.

The Galenic system that dominated medical thinking into the seventeenth century was based on the ancient Hippocratic tradition and on Aristotelian philosophy. The Greco-Roman physician Galen (A.D. 129–ca. 199) popularized a theory now known as the doctrine of the four humors—blood, phlegm, black bile, and yellow bile. The four humors corresponded with the four elements of ancient Greek philosophy, air, water, earth, and fire, which in turn were associated with the qualities of dry, moist, cold, and hot. Illness was thought to result from an alteration in the balance among the humors. Therapy was thus directed toward restoring the balance to achieve health.

With the coming of the Scientific Revolution, a new generation of medical thinkers began to question traditional doctrines and develop a new philosophy of medicine. For example, the Belgian surgeon and anatomist Andreas Vesalius (1514–1564) explored the human body through dissection and presented a more accurate view of its structure. Dr. William Harvey (1578–1657) challenged the medical community's tenets concerning the heartbeat, pulse, and movement of blood when he proved that it circulated continuously through the body.

KENNETH McKENZIE (?–1755)

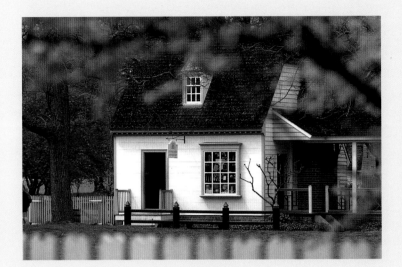

This apothecary shop was reconstructed on Palace green on the site where Dr. Kenneth McKenzie practiced during the 1740s and 1750s. His extensive medical library reveals much about the body of available medical knowledge.

Dr. Kenneth McKenzie advertised his medical business in the *Virginia Gazette* in May 1745. He had married Joanna Tyler (a great-aunt of President John Tyler) in 1738[13] and the couple had three children. Anne married Dr. David Black from the Petersburg area, William became a doctor himself, and Mary died at the age of two months. Little else is known about McKenzie's early life and family except that a cousin with the same name lived across the James River in Surry, Virginia, and also practiced medicine.

Although nothing is known of Dr. McKenzie's education, he left an impressive medical library when he died on March 17, 1755. Of seventy-one titles listed in the inventory of his estate, sixty-three were medical books. More than 30 percent of the doctor's medical library was devoted to anatomy, surgery, and midwifery. He owned classics such as Hermann Boerhaave's *Chymistry,* John Ranby's *On Gunshot Wounds,* and Richard Mead's *On Smallpox,* along with books on pharmacy, chemistry, fevers, smallpox, and the general practice of medicine.

An Inventory of Dr. Kenneth McKenzie's Medical Library

Cooper's Anatomy
Hoadly on Respiration
Ranby on Gun Shot Wounds
Medicina Statica
London Dispensatory
Keill's Anatomy
Robinson on Diseases
Hippocrates Aphorisms
Prasagium Medicum
Anatomical figures No. 11
  with the Explanation
Douglas's Midwifery
Boerhaave's Chymistry
Winston's Anatomy
Heister's Surgery
Douglas's Lythotomy
Heister's Compendium
Astruc on Women &c. Vol. 5
James's Dispensatory
Shaw's Dispensatory
Freind's History of Physic
Garengeol's Surgery
Mead's Precepts
Chapman's Midwifery
Harvey's De Motu Cordis
Cheyne on Health
Cheyne on the Gout
Cheselden on the Stone
Cheselden on Anatomy
Wilson's Chymistry
Praxis Medica

Monroe's Anatomy
Mead on Poisons
State of Midwifery
Le Dran's Operations 2 Vols.
Saviard's Observations
Sharp's Critical Enquiry
Saint-Yves on the Eyes
Sharp's Surgery
Medical Essays
Medical Essays Edinburgh
Thomson on Dissecting
Hurlock on Dentition
Petit on the Bones
Mauriceau's Midwifery
Deventer's Midwifery
Van Swieten 8 Vols.
Hillary on the Small Pox
Robinson on Decays
Sydenham's Works
Baglivi
Pitcairne
Bellini
Lommius on Fevers
Mead on Small Pox
Modern Practice of Physic 2 Vols.
Wainewright on Non-Naturals
Freind on Fevers
Freind's Emmenologia
Shaw's Practice of Physic 2 Vols.
Arbuthnot on Air
Turner 4 Vols.

Applying the principles of mathematics and mechanics developed by Descartes (1596–1650), Leibniz (1646–1716), and Newton (1642–1727), later seventeenth-century physicians began to explain the workings of the body in terms of mechanical principles by comparing the body to machines. By the early eighteenth century, Hermann Boerhaave (1668–1738) of Leiden developed the first comprehensive system to emphasize mechanical explanations for physiological activities and pathological processes. This new system dominated medical thinking for the first half of the eighteenth century and was studied by several Williamsburg practitioners, including Doctors de Sequeyra, Gilmer, Pasteur, and Galt.

Boerhaave described the structure of the body as an aggregation of solids and fluids. The solids were composed of minute particles that combined to form fibers. Fibers intertwined to form vessels that contained circulating fluids. The fluids, aggregates of minute particles, were the source of the various humors. Boerhaave surmised that solid parts provided firmness and stability to the body, while hollow vessels created by the fibers provided the vehicle by which fluids moved about and mixed, separated, or changed according to hydrostatic, hydraulic, and mechanical laws. Diseases were a result of a malfunction in this system. Said Boerhaave, "The Person who can perform the several Actions proper to the human Body with Ease, Pleasure, and a certain Constancy, is said to be well; and that Condition of the Body is termed Health. But if he either cannot perform those Actions; or if he performs them but with Difficulty, Pain and sudden Weariness; he is then said to be ill: and that State of the Body is call'd a Disease."[14]

Boerhaave explained that the causes of disease were twofold. The remote causes were a compilation of a person's predisposition such as age, gender, constitution, and temperament, while the procatarctic causes excited the predisposing causes into action. Procatarctic causes were substances taken into the body like air, food, drink, medicine, or poison; the amount, kind, and quality of activity, rest, and emotions; the quality and quantity of materials the body retained and excreted; and anything that came into contact with the exterior of the body such as air, water, clothing, or lotions. Together, the remote and procatarctic causes comprised the trigger that set off symptoms of disease. In other words, a person who was predisposed to a particular illness but was not exposed to any inciting factors would not become ill, and vice versa.

Only when both factors acted simultaneously did changes occur among the humors and solids that resulted in disease. Fibers could become too relaxed and weak or too rigid and strong. The humors could increase or decrease in amount. Their movement in the body could be too fast or too slow. The quality of the humors could also be imperfect. Such changes would then cause mechanical malfunctions in the various systems and symptoms would appear. Treatment was directed toward relieving the symptoms and removing the most immediate factor(s) that had triggered the illness.

The main components of this theory, now called "solidism" to contrast it with the earlier "humoralism," remained intact until William Cullen (1710–1790) proposed his theory. Cullen, who became a professor of medicine at Edinburgh University in 1766, theorized that the nervous system controlled and balanced tensions between the humors and the solids. The phenomena of disease, or symptoms, reflected varying degrees of contraction ranging from complete relaxation to excessive irritation and spasm in the network of blood vessels and nerves throughout the body. Even though Cullen proposed a new theory to explain the disease processes, like Boerhaave, he still directed treatment at the symptoms.

Diagnosis

Cullen realized, however, that it was difficult to distinguish among many disorders when their external appearances or symptoms were so much alike. "But as disorders different in their nature require different, and sometimes even opposite remedies, it becomes a matter of the greatest importance, that those practising Physic, should distinguish for a certainty each disorder from any other."[15] To this end, in 1769 Cullen published a nosology, a classification of diseases, to assist students and practitioners in diagnosis. Over the previous fifty years, other physicians had developed their own classifications based on each author's general theory of disease, but individual physicians still had to interpret a patient's symptoms in order to diagnose the condition.

Verbal interaction between doctor and patient was especially important for interpreting clues about the patient's condition. In the 1758 edition of *The General Practice of Physic*, Richard Brookes (fl. 1750s) wrote, "It will be therefore necessary to enquire into the Age, Sex, Structure, and

Habit of the Body, or the acquired Habit and Strength of the Patient, and whether he has an hereditary Disposition to this or that Disease."[16] Brookes continued that it "is likewise proper to know . . . whether the Vessels are slender and numerous, or large and few. . . . Regard is also to be had to the Colour of the Face and Skin. A fair, florid, and clear Complexion, show the Purity and Pellucidness of the lymphatic Fluids."[17] Without a healthy color, conditions, particularly of the liver, might develop.

Of special diagnostic interest was the state of the pulse and the condition of the body's excretions, particularly the urine. The pulse was a measure of the patient's overall strength of constitution. Strength and vigor shown by "Motion and Impulse of the Fluids . . . [indicate] great Hopes of recovering Health."[18] The regularity of the body's excretions was an integral part of good health. Any excretion—urine, sweat, semen, tears, mucous—that was judged to be "too plentiful, defective or suppressed . . . [could indicate] various Disorders" ranging from intestinal to respiratory complaints.[19] Cullen used a specific test involving mucous to determine if a patient suffered a catarrh (a cold) or the more serious phthisis (consumption of the lungs). He stated that normally sputum brought up from the lungs would float when dropped into water; if, however, the substance expectorated was pus, which was denser, it would sink.[20]

Diet also affected the general health of the patient. Too gross and heavy a diet would overtax the body's organs and produce obstructions in the digestive tract.

Not only was the condition of the body observed and assessed, so was the patient's mental state, as "there is a wonderful Connexion between the Mind and the Body." Brookes continued, "A greater Tensity and Mobility of the Fibres and Solids disposes the Mind to *Anger;* whereas a Laxity . . . [shows] the Person to be dispirited, timid and fearful."[21] The overtaxed and hyperactive mind was "subject to various Passions and Commotions" and could be cured only with difficulty.[22]

Williamsburg doctors often used these diagnostic techniques, which were by no means foolproof, to identify a variety of illnesses. Many Old World ailments were common in the Tidewater, among them smallpox, measles, and influenza, to name only three. Williamsburg physicians were well versed in recognizing and treating such conditions. Environment and geography often determined which ailments were more frequent or more

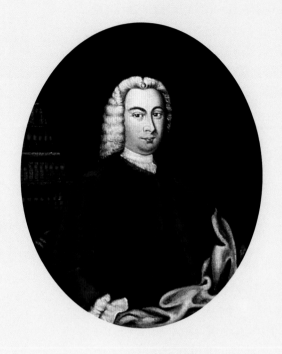

Dr. John de Sequeyra received his medical degree in 1739 from the University of Leiden in Holland. During his fifty years in Williamsburg, Dr. de Sequeyra became the first visiting physician to the Public Hospital. Courtesy, Winterthur Museum.

plaints often carried over into the spring when the intermittent fevers returned. Summertime complaints included dysentery and whooping cough.[24]

In a separate account, the doctor kept a record by household of the effects of the 1747–1748 smallpox epidemic. He noted which households were struck, the numbers that were taken ill, and how many recovered or died. In many instances, he recorded whether the patient was a family member or a slave. The list included the college and Governor Gooch's household as well as prominent town residents from the Geddy, Wetherburn, Tarpley, Prentis, and McKenzie families. This record provides early population statistics for Williamsburg.

De Sequeyra was the first visiting physician to the "Public Hospital for Persons of Insane and Disordered Minds" that opened in Williamsburg on October 12, 1773. Modeled on similar institutions in Europe, the hospital was the first facility of its kind in the colonies. Dr. de Sequeyra oversaw new admissions and provided the health care for the patients.

Thomas Jefferson credited de Sequeyra with introducing the tomato, a fruit formerly thought to be poisonous, into Virginia. Along with eighty-three other well-known Virginians, the physician subscribed annually for eight years to a prize for producing the best wine in the colony.

Little is known of de Sequeyra's personal life in Williamsburg. There is no evidence of marriage or children. He owned two slaves, two horses, and a four-wheeled post chaise. On June 18, 1772, de Sequeyra signed a seven-year lease with Williamsburg merchant William Goodson for three rooms at the east end of a large dwelling house on the south side of Duke of Gloucester Street, along with some of the adjoining lands and outbuildings, part of the cellar, half of the garden, and use of the well, all for five shillings plus £30 annually.[25] When he died in early 1795 at the age of eighty-three, the *Virginia Gazette and General Advertiser* described John de Sequeyra as having been "an eminent famous physician."[26]

John de Sequeyra was born in London to a well-to-do medical family of Portuguese Jewish descent. He left England in 1736 to pursue medicine at the University of Leiden in Holland where he reportedly studied with Boerhaave and almost certainly with Boerhaave's successor, Jerome David Gaub. De Sequeyra received a doctor's degree in medicine on February 3, 1739.

Dr. de Sequeyra sailed for Virginia in 1745 and settled in Williamsburg, where he was highly regarded by both colleagues and fellow citizens. Among his patients was George Washington's stepdaughter, Patsy Custis, whom he treated for epilepsy in 1769.

Perhaps an early interest in his newly adopted homeland prompted de Sequeyra's accounting of the illnesses he observed each year in and around Williamsburg from 1745 to 1781. The physician noted that many conditions recurred during the same seasons in every year. For example, he wrote in September 1745 that "Fall produced intermittent Fevers,"[23] a statement he repeated nearly every year. Autumn in Williamsburg also generated dysentery, worms in children, measles, mumps, and whooping cough. Winter gave rise to respiratory problems such as pleurisy and colds as well as smallpox and scarlet fever. These com-

serious, which less so. Typhus and smallpox were more prevalent in towns than in rural areas. Yellow fever occurred more frequently in coastal towns.

Colonial doctors traveled to patients' homes when illness became serious, thus establishing the private residence as the infirmary. In Europe, public hospitals were overcrowded with the sick poor and lacked effective sanitary arrangements. As a consequence, diseases spread quite rapidly among patients. By the mid-seventeenth century, Virginia witnessed some of the first smallpox pesthouses. Temporary facilites to care for the military during the Revolution existed in a few places in Tidewater Virginia. In Williamsburg, the vacated Governor's Palace and the Wren Building at the College of William and Mary were used for that purpose.

Therapy

Regimen was the first stage of a planned system of therapy, which used the natural habits of the body to reverse the course of disease. According to an eighteenth-century European authority, the cure of a disease was "to be attempted first by a proper diet and regimen, and secondly, by the direct use of medicines peculiarly adapted to the particular symptoms or nature of the case."[27] Patients expected practitioners to provide a miracle medication that relieved their complaints and returned their body to health. However, a wise physician knew that physic "can do nothing but remove Impediments, resolve Obstructions, cut off and tear away *Excrescences* and Superfluities, and reduce Nature to its primitive Order."[28] In other words, healing depended on nature with help from the doctor.

Diet, exercise, and air quality constituted the "regimen" for maintaining health and treating disease. Regimen decreased the severity of the symptoms and prepared the body to benefit from the remedies. Because food sustained the body during health and illness, an appropriate diet was important. "Diseases are always to be cured by their *Contraries*, the *high Diet* by the *low*, the *hot* by the *cool*, the *sapid* by the *insipid*, the *thick* and gross by the *thin* and poor."[29] A certain amount of exercise was essential to maintain the correct strength and elasticity within the fibers and proper circulation of the fluids. Riding on horseback was regarded as the best activity to restore health; walking most advantageous for preserving it. Finally, air must be "pure and sweet, void of all bad Exhalations, neither too hot, nor cold, nor dry, nor moist."[30]

WILLIAM PASTEUR (1737?–1791)

William Pasteur[31] was the only son of
Jean Pasteur, a Swiss Huguenot who
emigrated to the colonies in 1700,
and Martha Harris. William's parents
had died by the mid-1740s, and Commissary Dawson of the College of
William and Mary became his
guardian. Although nothing is known
of William's early education, his
guardian may have seen that he
received grammar school education
at the college. In 1752, Pasteur completed a medical apprenticeship with
Dr. George Gilmer, Sr., and then continued his medical studies at St.
Thomas's Hospital in London.

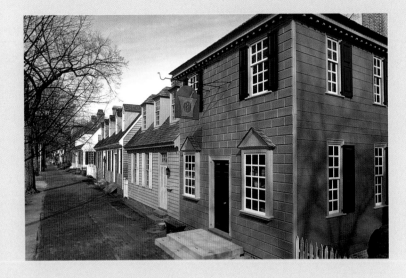

By 1760, Pasteur had returned to Williamsburg, established a
practice, and opened an apothecary shop on the east end of Duke of
Gloucester Street. He "was well thought of as a doctor."[32] About that
time, he married Elizabeth Stith, daughter of the president of William
and Mary. They had one child, William Stith Pasteur, who was born in
November 1762 and died young.[33]

Dr. Pasteur formed a partnership with Dr. John Minson Galt in
April 1775. The *Virginia Gazette* announced, "They intend practising
Physic and Surgery to their fullest Extent; and that they intend
also . . . to keep full and complete Assortments of Drugs and Medicines, which they will endeavour to procure of the very best Quality,
and will take Care to have them fresh by making several Importations
in the Year."[34] In that same year, Pasteur was elected mayor of
Williamsburg. The medical partnership dissolved in 1778 and Pasteur
sold his share of the business to Galt.

In his "retirement," Dr. Pasteur made a dramatic and surprising
career change by becoming an oyster merchant! He was appointed a
coroner in York County in 1780. In 1790, Pasteur became director of
the Public Hospital for the Insane, but held the position only briefly,
possibly due to ill health. At his death in 1791, Pasteur left instruc-
tions to sell his Beaverdam plantation on the James River, including
crops, livestock, and other assets—except slaves—to pay his debts.

Today, Dr. William Pasteur's
reconstructed apothecary shop on
Duke of Gloucester Street is open
to visitors with tickets. The four
authors of this book interpret
medical history on the site.

After regimen, the second stage of therapy involved prescribing various medications. Surviving newspaper advertisements provide insight into the wide variety of chemicals, minerals, and botanicals that were used in pharmaceuticals. Dr. Pasteur placed the following advertisement in the *Virginia Gazette* in September 1769:

Just imported from *LONDON*, in the *Experiment*, Capt. *Hamlin*, and to be *SOLD*, at the subscriber's shop, in *WILLIAMSBURG*,

A LARGE and compleat assortment of DRUGS and MEDICINES, both chymical and galenical, consisting of antimony, alum, aloes of all sorts, æther, borax, quicksilver, camphire, castor, cochineal, best Jesuits-drops, and bark, ipecacuanha, jalap, sarsaparilla and China roots, essence of lemons and bergamot, manna, calomel, red and white precipitate, calcined mercury, magnesia alba, best Turkey and India rhubarb, spermaceti, oil of turpentine, volatile spirits, and salts of all sorts. Also cinnamon, cloves, mace, nutmegs, ginger, black pepper, sago, salop, candied figs, prunes, white and brown candies, orange chips, currants, best jar raisins, capers, olives and anchovies, best Durham flower of mustard, common and Clay's best sallad oil, verdigrease, vermilion, Prussian blue, gold and silver leaf, neat smelling bottles, with cases; ivory syringes, Greenhough's tincture for the teeth and gums, ditto for the tooth ach, tooth brushes, pumice and rotten stone, best lancets, court plaister, Agard's pills, much esteemed for the rheumatism, and Blackrie's lixivium for the gravel; also British rock oil, Bateman's and Stoughton's drops, Godfrey's and Trueman's cordials, Daffy's and Squire's elixir, essence of water dock, elixir bardana, Turlington's balsam and balsam of honey, Dr. James's fever powders, Anderson's and Lockyer's pills, and Mrs. Rednapp's fit drops, &c. &c. &c.

The subscriber having had but very few MEDICINES in his shop before this order came to hand, will now be able to furnish his friends and customers with every thing fresh and genuine. Gentlemen practitioners and others may depend on being supplied at a very low advance, by their humble servant,

WILLIAM PASTEUR.[35]

Medications were divided into categories according to their effects. Some ingredients such as rhubarb, prunes, and magnesia alba (magnesium carbonate) were used as laxatives. Alum and oil of turpentine were styptics that stopped bleeding. Ready-made medicines like Bateman's drops for coughs and Dr. James's Fever Powders, a mercuric compound used to treat

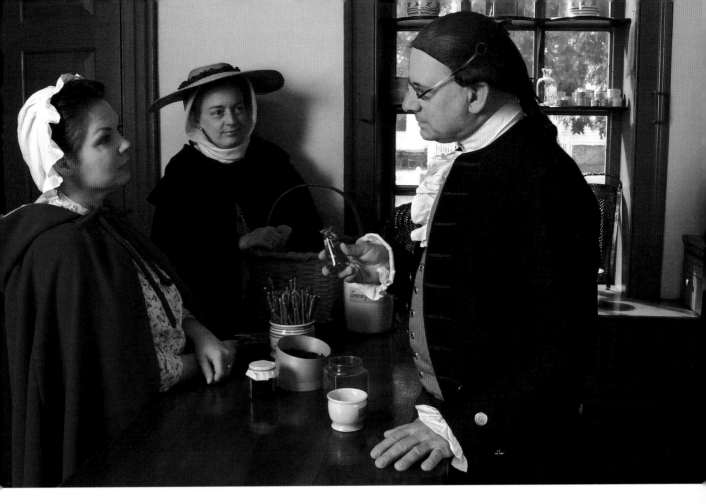

Governor Botetourt, were also sold. Patent medicines were available in Williamsburg at apothecary shops, the post office, and Catherine

Rathell's millinery shop. Since medications were not regulated, it was not necessary to consult a physician before buying them from an apothecary. However, opium and other medications may have been dispensed at the discretion of the apothecary due to the potential for toxic effects.

The advertisement also listed sundries with multiple applications. Cinnamon, cloves, and ginger were used, respectively, to treat gas, toothaches, and nausea, and in cooking. Crushed cochineal beetles provided a red powder for dyeing fabric, to use in cosmetics, and to color food and drugs.

Doctors prescribed medicines based on the patient's disorder and associated symptoms. Some items were given more frequently than others. Dr. Galt's account book indicates that laxatives were among the most frequently prescribed medications. Entries in most accounts, however, do not denote the specific medication administered or sold and provide little if any information about the diagnosis. Medicines mentioned by name include ipecac, Peruvian bark, and opium.

As noted in Dr. de Sequeyra's records, dysentery was a problem in Williamsburg. The characteristic symptoms, cramping and diarrhea, were believed by some to be caused by eating unripe summer fruit that fermented in the stomach. Attempting to remove the stomach contents by inducing vomiting with a preparation of ipecac (*Cephaelis ipecacuanha*) was considered an appropriate treatment. Later, it was discovered that there are two types of dysentery, bacillary dysentery, caused by bacteria, and amebic dysentery, caused by a protozoan, a one-celled organism. Today, severe cases of amebic dysentery can be treated with emetine, a derivative of ipecac, and other medications.

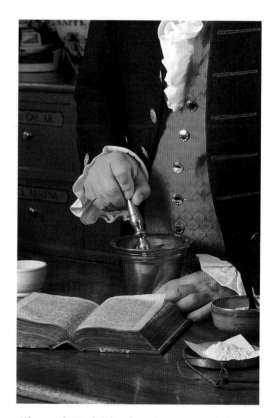

Dr. de Sequeyra also noted intermitting fever, an eighteenth-century term for malaria, in the Tidewater area. Doctors prescribed cinchona bark (*Cinchona officinalis*) for this condition. In 1820, it was discovered that cinchona contains quinine. The use of quinine in today's medicine has been largely replaced with synthetic products, although it is still used in some malaria cases that are resistant to modern synthetic anti-malarial drugs.

Opium (*Papaver somniferum*) was prescribed for pain, diarrhea, and severe coughing. Today, derivatives of this plant are given for the same purposes. Numerous other drugs available in the eighteenth century could relieve symptoms as well. In

(Above and opposite) Apothecaries compounded most of the medicines that they prescribed. A wide variety of imported botanicals, chemicals, minerals, and other ingredients were mixed according to the directions in professional pharmacy texts. Dry ingredients were weighed and liquids were measured using graduated glass cylinders. The finished products included infusions, tinctures, pills, and ointments.

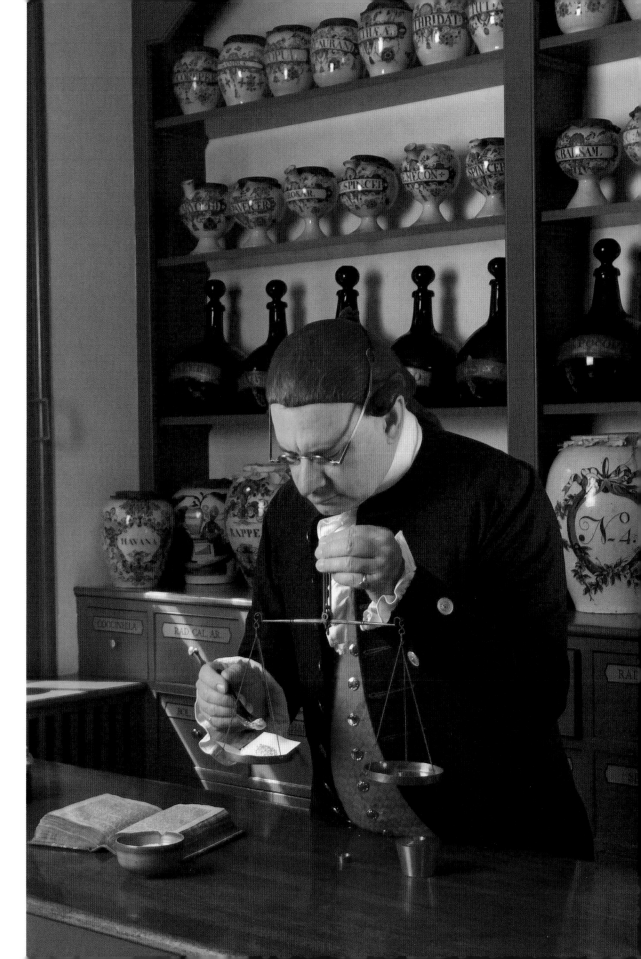

the 1760s, Dr. Anton Störck from Vienna promoted autumn crocus (*Colchicum autumnale*) as a treatment for gout.[36] The plant contains colchicine, which is still used for that purpose. Purple foxglove (*Digitalis purpurea*) was prescribed in the late eighteenth century by doctors to treat dropsy (edema). It was discovered later that in some cases dropsy is a symptom of congestive heart failure. The active principle, digitoxin, is used today in the treatment of congestive heart failure and other cardiac disorders. Additional medications whose applications have remained largely unchanged since the eighteenth century include chalk as an antacid, calamine for skin irritations, senna (*Cassia acutifolia*) and castor oil as laxatives, and juniper oil as a diuretic.

Few eighteenth-century medications could actually cure a condition or inhibit the further development of a disease. An exception was scurvy, caused by the lack of ascorbic acid (vitamin C). Eighteenth-century pharmacy books recommended an assortment of citrus fruits that were later proven to contain vitamin C. Although scurvy was not a significant problem in Williamsburg, Dr. Galt treated at least one case.

The extent to which syphilis was present in the area is not known. Records indicate that some of Dr. Galt's patients were diagnosed with venereal disease. Mercurial salts such as calomel were prescribed for patients with syphilis. Modern studies indicate that mercury may inhibit the growth of the microorganism that causes syphilis.[37]

The formulas for preparing medications were published in professional pharmacy texts called pharmacopoeias and dispensatories. In 1764, Dr. Pasteur purchased a copy of *The New Dispensatory* for John Galt. Of the sixty-three medical titles in Dr. Kenneth McKenzie's library, three were dispensatories. Such texts were an important part of a practitioner's library because they contained general advice on preparing medications and dosage. They also provided background information on the theory and practice of pharmacy. Some texts, such as *The New Dispensatory*, gave advice on preparing medicines for the poor.

Colonial apothecaries depended on imported supplies to make their medications. Most ingredients in British pharmacy books were not native to the colonies. Dr. Pasteur's advertisement illustrated his dependence on imported supplies since he indicated that his inventory of medicines was low prior to the arrival of his latest shipment. Dr. James Carter's business accounts for 1752–1774 are typical. During that time, he purchased drugs from more than a dozen suppliers in Liverpool, Bristol, and London, England. In 1755, Carter bought drugs and equipment from the estate of former competitor Dr. McKenzie. Two years later, he purchased drugs from the estate of Dr. Gilmer, Sr.

The author of *Every Man his own Doctor* addressed the cost of importing drugs when promoting his domestic medical guide. In the third edition (1736), he noted:

The Remedies I have prescrib'd, are almost all of our own Growth, there being no more than 5 or 6 foreign Medicines; and they so very cheap, that if I happen not to cure my Patient, I am sure I shan't ruin him. . . . Neither do I ransack the Universe for outlandish Drugs, which must waste and decay in a long Voyage; nor import the Sweepings of the Shops, which I am sure are decay'd but; am content to do all my Execution with the Weapons of our own Country.[38]

"Ransacking the Universe" for drugs was an apt metaphor. The ingredients that reached Williamsburg via British merchants came from all over the world. Rhubarb roots were imported from Turkey and Russia. Opium came primarily

This 1757 excerpt from Dr. James Carter's invoice book lists medicines that he purchased from the estate of Dr. George Gilmer, Sr. The total purchase price was £544.

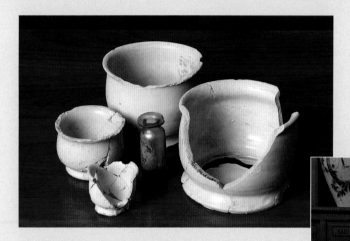

Dr. George Gilmer was a very successful Williamsburg professional in both medicine and politics.
His date of birth is not known,[39] and nothing is
known of his early life. He received medical
schooling at the University of Edinburgh and was
established in Williamsburg by 1731.

Records indicate that Gilmer married two, possibly three, times.[40] His
first recorded marriage in Williamsburg was to Mary Peachy Walker,
daughter of a former partner, Dr. Thomas Walker of King and Queen
County, Virginia. They had two sons, Peachy, born in 1737, and George,
Jr., born in 1742, who followed his father into medicine. Both sons lived
full lives. Mary died October 1, 1745, after a severe but short illness. On
December 11, 1745, Dr. Gilmer married Harrison Blair, daughter of
Archibald Blair and sister of the Honorable John Blair, president of the
College of William and Mary. They also had two sons, John, born on
April 26, 1748, and William, born on May 22, 1753, who died eight days
later. Gilmer wrote in his family bible, "The poor babe died the 30th,
and was buried on the 31st, by the Commissary, in a grave so close to
my dear former wife, that his coffin touched hers."[41]

Gilmer served as justice of the peace from the late 1730s to the 1750s
and as sheriff in the 1740s. He was elected mayor of Williamsburg in
December 1754 after enticing voters with a hearty bout of drinking to
help him win votes against John Randolph. Gilmer was also part owner of
the Raleigh Tavern.

Numerous advertisements in the *Virginia Gazette* indicate that Dr. Gilmer
sold the same variety of items as his competitors. At one point, he corrected
rumors of an unsuccessful business and his supposed death, strongly stating
in the local paper that the rumors must have been started by a rival doctor.

Artifacts from the Gilmer site
include gallipots, a glass vial, and a
blue-and-white delftware apothecary
jar. In 1957 and 1988, excavations
on Dr. Gilmer's property near
Palace green revealed five trash
pits filled with household and
apothecary discards from 1735 to
1737. Ointment pots and English
delftware drug jars, pill tiles, large
bottles, or carboys, and other
pharmaceutical bottles were
uncovered. This discovery is the
most complete accumulation of
mid-eighteenth-century apothecary
items recovered in Williamsburg
and affords a comprehensive view
of storage vessels used by
colonial practitioners.

from Egypt and Persia. Senna was grown in Persia, Syria, and Arabia. Licorice came from England, cinchona and ipecac from Peru. By contrast, only a few native Virginia plant remedies—sassafras, ginseng, and Virginia snakeroot—were recognized in professional pharmacy books.

Monopolies increased the prices of some items. For instance, the Dutch had a monopoly on spices from the East Indies and camphor from Japan. Drugs that were expensive or difficult to collect were especially vulnerable to adulteration by import companies to increase profits. Dr. Pasteur made a point in his advertisement that his drugs were fresh and genuine. Chemistry books, purchasing guides, and dispensatories offered advice on this issue as it was very difficult to identify adulterated drugs. Since Jamaica pepper oil had a similar aroma and flavor, it was mixed with the more costly clove oil. Some companies added chalk to the white lead used in eye ointments for higher profits. To combat this problem, one author suggested deleting nonessential drugs from pharmacy books, thus removing the temptation to sell costly imitations.

Eighteenth-century authors compared their medications with ancient and medieval medicines, perhaps gaining a sense of satisfaction that progress had been achieved. While twenty-first-century practitioners may find some problems with these medications, colonial doctors viewed their drugs as a product of traditional practice and modern science. Drug therapy was not the solution for every disorder, however, and additional treatment such as bloodletting was considered necessary in some cases.

Bloodletting

Defined as "the Puncture, Incision, or Aperture of some Blood-Vessel, in order to take out of it such a Quantity of Blood as is judg'd proper and convenient,"[42] bloodletting is probably the most often talked about yet least understood of all eighteenth-century medical treatments. Phlebotomy or venesection, opening a vein with a sharp, pointed, steel instrument, was the most common technique and the only one mentioned in Williamsburg accounts that have survived. The French or thumb lancet was the usual phlebotomy instrument. In addition, there were spring lancets to puncture a vein to a specific depth using the force of a steel spring, and fleams primarily for veterinary practice but also used on humans.

Occasionally carried out on the hand, foot, temples, neck, or under

DRUG JARS

Popular for storing medications in the seventeenth and eighteenth centuries, English delftware drug jars were mass produced at large manufacturing centers in Bristol, Liverpool, London, and Glasgow. Each piece was thrown on a potter's wheel, fired, thickly coated with a lead glaze that contained tin oxide, and fired a second time. The resulting opaque white glaze provided a good background for labels and artwork. Some eighteenth-century English decorations were simple, while others depicted cherubs, tassels, flowers, songbirds, and baskets of fruit. The characteristic blue color in many designs was created by adding cobalt to the glaze. It was the preferred color in large-scale production because it withstood the high firing temperatures better than other colors.

Some containers featured Latin labels, the prefix denoting the variety of medication. "S" indicated *syrupus,* a saturated solution of water and sugar, "C" meant *conservæ,* a sugar-based mixture, and "U" represented *unguentum,* an ointment.

Tastes were changing by the late eighteenth century. The demand for delftware drug jars was declining as apothecaries opted for the more fashionable creamware. Nevertheless, some demand continued for utilitarian objects made of delft, such as storage containers and ointment pots. These items were produced well into the next century.

The evolution in style of English delft apothecary shelfware is evident in these antique syrup containers. Left to right: back view, mid-eighteenth century, front view, mid-eighteenth century featuring the Latin name for syrup of violets, front view of a seventeenth-century vessel labeled syrup of raspberries. Note the changes in the cherub pattern and the design and location for the spout.

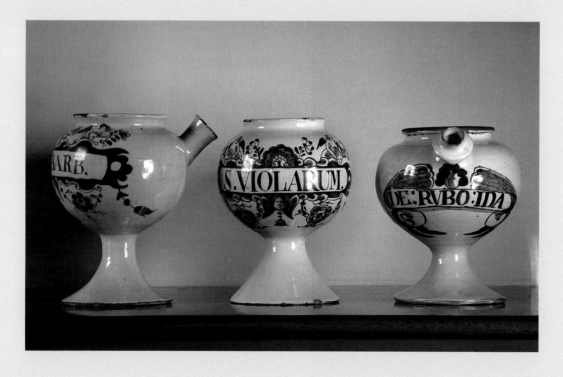

the tongue, bloodletting was usually performed in one of the three veins that lie inside the elbow. After puncturing a vein, the blood was collected in a special bleeding bowl or other receptacle. The blood flow was then stopped with compression and elevation.

Scarification removed blood through a series of small incisions in the skin where veins and arteries were not in danger of being cut. The incisions could be made with a lancet or scarificator, a small brass box fitted with twelve to twenty blades that penetrated the skin simultaneously at a predetermined depth. The cuts were usually covered with a cupping glass in which a partial vacuum had been created by burning lint or tow (flax) inside or by holding it over a flame. The vacuum helped draw blood from the capillaries into the cup. Sometimes scarification was performed without cupping.

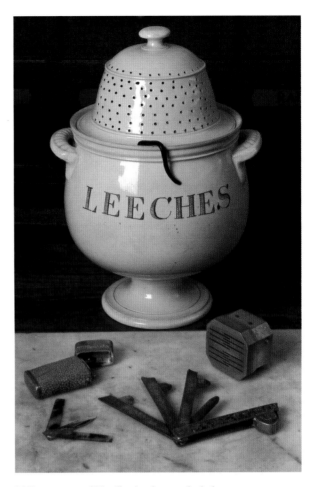

Different types of bleeding implements include *(counterclockwise from the top)* **leeches, a lancet, fleam, and scarificator.**

Leeches were also used to draw blood. Approximately 650 species exist around the world. *Hirudo medicinalis,* the species most commonly used, is native to freshwaters in Central and Northern Europe. In the eighteenth century, leeches were used on parts of the body where the lancet could not easily be applied, particularly on "young Children, whose Veins seem too small to admit of Puncture by an Instrument with safety."[43]

Doctors prescribed bloodletting mainly for inflammatory conditions characterized by redness, swelling, pain, and heat. It was also used for plethora "where the vessels are overfilled with a thick dense blood."[44] In

1774, Dr. William Buchan wrote a thorough description of when blood-letting should occur:

Bleeding is proper at the beginning of all inflammatory fevers, as pleurisies, peripneumonies, &c. It is likewise proper in all topical inflammations, as those of the intestines, womb, bladder, stomach, kidnies, throat, eyes, &c.; as also in the asthma, sciatic pains, coughs, head-achs, rheumatisms, the apoplexy, epilepsy and bloody-flux. After falls, blows, bruises, or any violent hurt received either externally or internally, bleeding is necessary. It is likewise necessary for persons who have had the misfortune to be strangled, drowned, suffocated with foul air, the fumes of metals, or the like.[45]

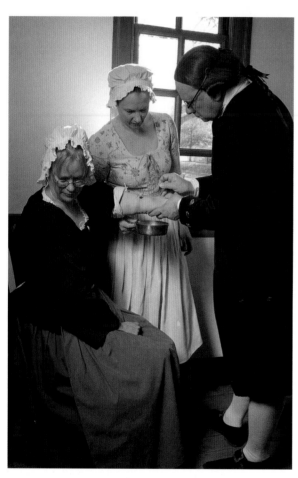

To bleed in the arm, a linen tourniquet is applied above the elbow and the patient is given a wooden dowel to grip. Holding the lancet between his thumb and forefinger, the doctor carefully penetrates the vein, then immediately flicks the blade upward to enlarge the opening.

The amount of blood removed varied with the patient's disorder, age, gender, strength, lifestyle, constitution, and the judgment of the bloodletter.

Surgery

There are few surviving records to provide clues about the surgical work performed in eighteenth-century Williamsburg. The word "surgery," translated from ancient Greek, literally means "hand-work." Beyond a handful of cases mentioning venesection, the most common procedure recorded was dental extraction.

By the 1740s, people had increased access to new developments in dentistry. The anatomy and pathology of the teeth were

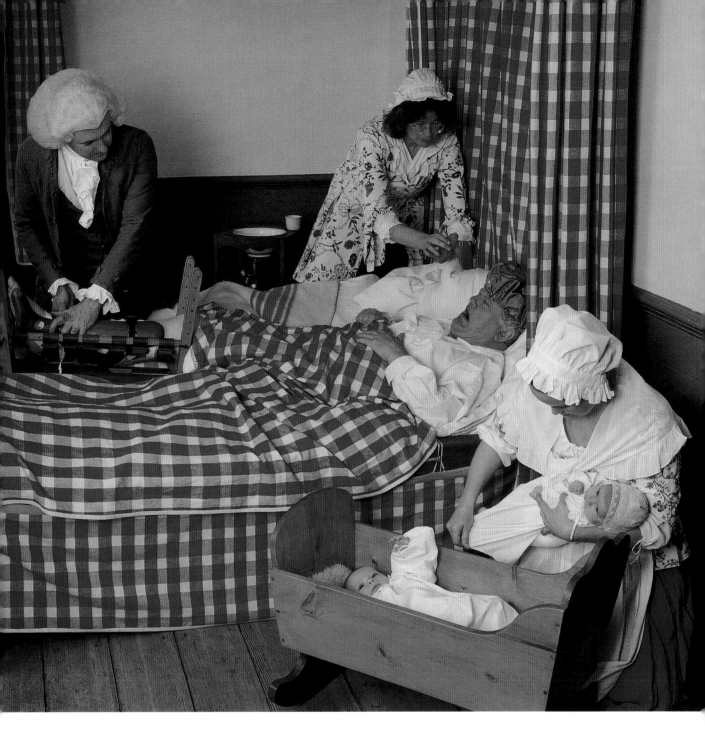

The fracture box, invented by surgeon James Rae, was useful when treating compound fractures. The instrument allowed the attending surgeon to inspect and dress wounds without moving the limb. The patient was treated at home where family members could provide daily care.

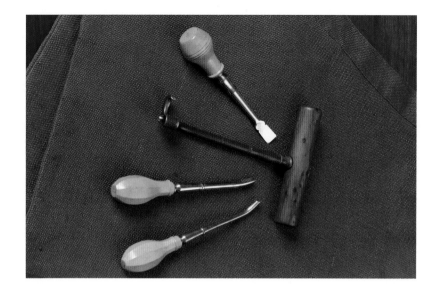

Instruments for extracting and excavating teeth. *Top to bottom*: dental chisel to break an impacted tooth, tooth key for lower molar extraction, and two "goat's foot" elevators for lifting out teeth and bone.

better known, causes and prevention of decay were more clearly under-stood, and the materials used to reconstruct and replace teeth had improved.

Surgeon-dentist John Baker, who claimed to have worked in Britain, Holland, France, Jamaica, and New England, moved to Williamsburg in 1771. Initially, Baker worked where he lived, renting space at the Maupin House located near Market Square, and later purchasing the Blair prop-erty nearby. Baker advertised an extensive range of services in 1772:

Mr. *BAKER*, Surgeon Dentist,

Begs Leave to inform the Gentry that he is now at Mr. Maupin's in Williams-burg, and will wait on them on receiving their commands. He cures the SCURVY in the GUMS, be it ever so bad; first cleans and scales the Teeth from that corro-sive, tartarous, gritty Substance which hinders the Gums from growing, infects the Breath, and is one of the principal Causes of the Scurvy, which, if not timely pre-vented, eats away the Gums, so that many Peoples Teeth fall out fresh. He pre-vents Teeth from growing rotten, keeps such as are decayed from becoming worse, even at old Age, makes the Gums grow up firm to the Teeth, and renders them white and beautiful. He fills up, with Lead or Gold, those that are hollow, so as to render them useful; it prevents the Air from getting into them, which aggravates the Pain. He transplants natural Teeth from one Person to another, which will be as firm in the Jaw as if they originally grew there, without any Ligament. He makes and fixes artificial Teeth with the greatest Exactness and Nicety, without Pain or the least Inconvenience, so that they may eat, drink, or sleep, with them in their Mouths as natural Ones, from which they cannot be discovered by the sharpest Eye. He displaces Teeth and Stumps, after the best and easiest Methods, be they ever so deep sunk into the Socket of the Gums. He has given sufficient Proof of his Abilities in this Art to the principal Nobility, Gentry, and others, of Great Britain, France, Ireland, Holland, *and other principal Places in* Europe *and* America; *also to upwards of two Thousand Persons in* New York *and* Boston.[46]

George Washington paid Baker to repair his teeth and ivory dentures. He also purchased various cleaning items. Dr. Baker advertised a tooth powder that prevented scurvy in the gums and cleaned the teeth. A leading Parisian doctor, Pierre Fauchard (1678–1761), recommended a dentifrice of pumice and alum to be finely powdered and sifted and applied with a slightly dampened sea sponge. Fauchard advised against cleaning the teeth with pieces of cloth or linen or with horsehair brushes, noting that people who cleaned in this manner "did so in ignorance."[47]

Toothbrushes and powdered dentifrices were also available from non-medical sources, among them Williamsburg milliner Catherine Rathell, who advertised ivory and tortiseshell toothpicks, toothpick cases, tooth-

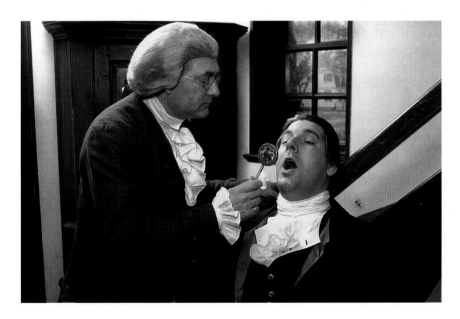

A surgeon holds a mirror for a patient while explaining a dental procedure.

39

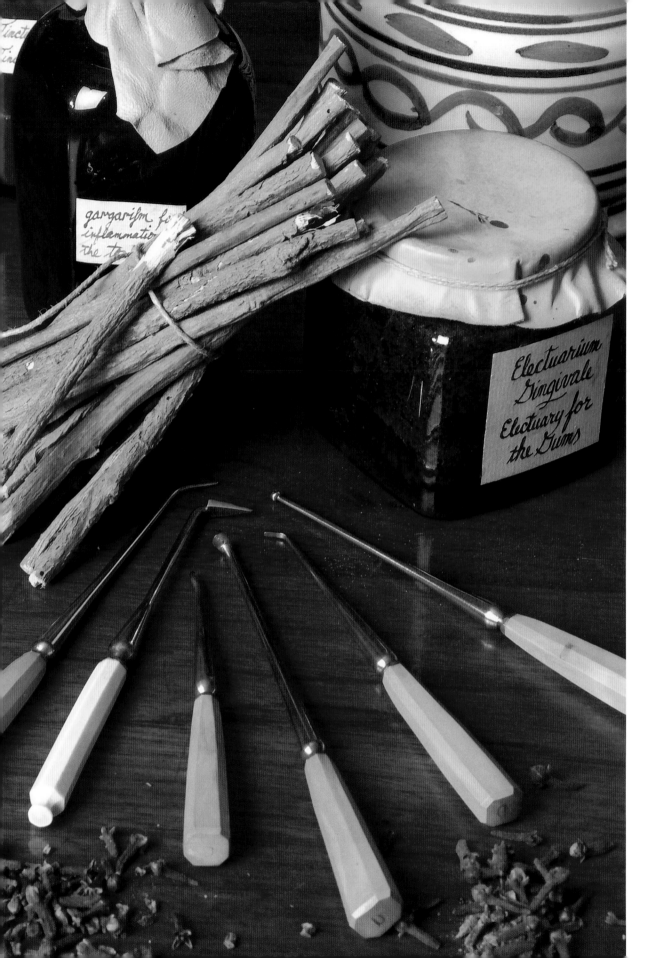

gargarism for
inflammation of
the t...

Electuarium
Gingivale
Electuary for
the Gums

brushes, and a pearl dentifrice for cleaning and preserving both teeth and gums.[48] Home remedy books recommended ground cuttlefish bone, cinnamon, cream of tartar, alum, or lemon juice. Improper dental hygiene resulted in frequent tooth extraction at all levels of society.

Baker and other surgeons in the colonies were further influenced by practitioners in Europe. A major leader in dental surgery, John Hunter (1728–1793) of Scotland, experimented with various surgical and dental techniques, including the transplantation of human teeth from one mouth to another. This procedure was attempted as an alternative to dentures, but often it was not successful.

References to other operations are harder to come by, even though they must have occurred. In 1769, John Galt and Andrew Anderson advertised in Williamsburg as apothecaries, surgeons, and man-midwives. When William Pasteur and John Galt notified the public of their partnership in 1775, they announced, "*John M. Galt* shall pay his particular attention to surgery . . . but will be advised and assisted by *W. Pasteur* in all difficult cases."[49]

Williamsburg doctors owned a number of surgical books and various instruments. The texts covered everything from bandaging to cesarean section, and a number of prominent authors were represented. Dr. McKenzie owned instruments for amputating, trepanning (removing a circular disk of bone from the skull), and lithotomy (removing bladder stones). The inventory of Dr. Alexander Middleton, a Tory who fled Williamsburg at the beginning of the Revolution, had tools for amputation, trepanning, lithotomy, couching (a form of cataract surgery), midwifery, and "For the teeth."[50] An inventory of Dr. Galt's implements has not survived, although he advertised in 1774 for the return of a lost chair box "containing sundry Wearing Apparel and SURGEONS INSTRUMENTS."[51] Even though doctors owned surgical apparatus and books that described their use, it should not be concluded that they performed certain operations.

The *Virginia Gazette* reported two instances of major operations that occurred in Williamsburg. Anthony Hay, a prominent Williamsburg businessman, died in 1770 of

Opposite: items for oral hygiene.
Left to right: "gargarism," or gargle of lemon juice, licorice roots (*Glycyrrhiza glabra*) that were chewed on one end to form a toothbrush, instruments for scraping and filling teeth, and "Electuarium Gingivale," a jellylike substance ingested for scurvy.

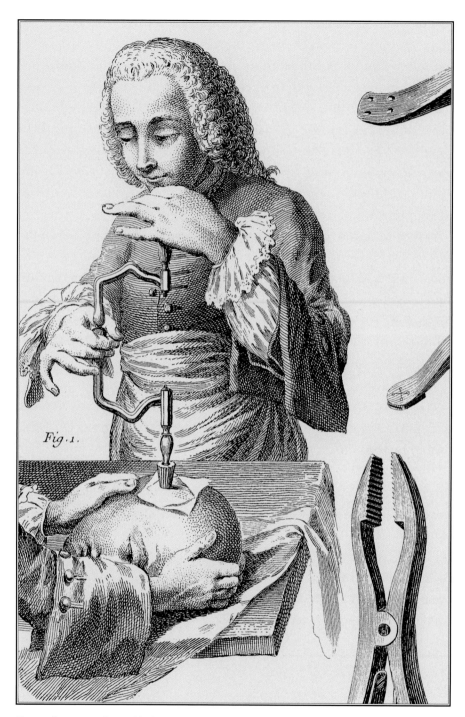

Trepanning was performed in fissures, fractures, and depressions of
the cranium in order to discharge fluid and remove any bone pressing
on the brain.

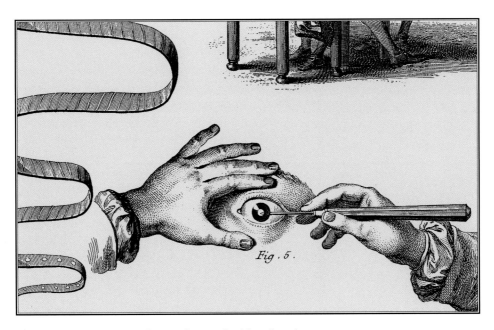

In Paris during the 1740s and 1750s, Jacques Daviel perfected a technique to extract cataracts instead of just couching them. His procedure continued to be used until laser surgery became the common method of treatment.

facial cancer. His obituary noted that Hay "underwent several severe operations, in his lip and face, for the disorder."[52] Most surgeons believed that surgical removal of the cancer was the only effective way to treat it. Even then, there was no guarantee the operation would be successful. According to the *Encyclopedia Britannica* (1771), cancers of the throat and palate were incurable; cancer of the lips was hard to cure.

The other operation, cataract couching, was performed by Dr. Graham. Among the sufferers he reportedly treated was Mrs. Cobb from Williamsburg who lost her sight due to cataracts on both eyes. The *Gazette* recounted that Dr. Graham couched her cataracts, and in less than five minutes she was said to have regained her sight.[53] Couching for cataracts meant only pushing the opacified lens away from the pupil of the eye. Unfortunately for Mrs. Cobb, the "success" of her operation was probably temporary.

Even though a variety of operations were available in the eighteenth century, the scope of surgery was limited. Because general anesthesia was

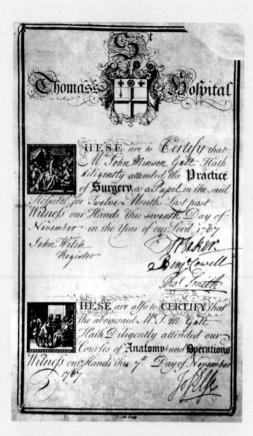

"St. Thomas's Hospital THESE are to Certify that Mr. John Galt Hath diligently attended the Practice of Surgery as a Pupil in the said Hospital for Twelve Months. Last past Witness our Hands this seventh Day of November in the Year of our Lord 1767 . . . THESE are also to CERTIFY that the abovesaid Mr. J. M. Galt Hath Diligently attended our Courses of Anatomy and Operations Witness our Hands this 7th Day of November 1767."

The son of Samuel Galt, a successful gold- and silver-smith, John Minson Galt became a prominent doctor, civic leader, and progenitor of a long line of medical practitioners. He was educated at the College of William and Mary. Following an apprenticeship in Williamsburg, Galt traveled to London where he earned certificates in theory and practice of physic (1767) from St. Thomas's Hospital, anatomy and surgery (1767) from Dr. Hugh Smith, and theory and practice of midwifery (1768) from Dr. Colin Mackenzie.

Galt returned to Williamsburg in early 1769 and married Judith Craig, daughter of silversmith Alexander Craig, on April 6. His granddaughter, Sally Galt, described him as being "rather low in stature, but very powerfully built; his complexion was ruddy—his eye was piercing." His character was described as upright and benevolent and possessing a generous kindness to the poor.[54] The Galts had six children, four of whom survived. Sons William and Alexander also became doctors. William apprenticed with his father, completed his medical education in Philadelphia, and eventually settled in Louisville, Kentucky. Alexander graduated from the College of William and Mary and studied medicine between 1792 and 1794 at Oxford University, in part with the renowned Sir Astley Cooper. He also "walked the wards" at Guy's and St. Thomas's Hospitals in London.

In September 1769, John Minson Galt announced his intention of "opening shop at the Brick House, opposite the Coffee House."[55] He merged his practice with that of his friend Dr. William Pasteur in April 1775. When Dr. Pasteur retired three years later, Galt paid £1,650 to acquire sole ownership of the thriving business.

Dr. Galt was a vestryman at Bruton Parish Church and served on the board of visitors at the college. He was also a Freemason and on the Williamsburg committee of safety. During the Revolutionary War, Galt acted as surgeon to the Continental Hospital in Williamsburg and later to the 15th Virginia Regiment. For a time, he held the position of surgeon general of Virginia.

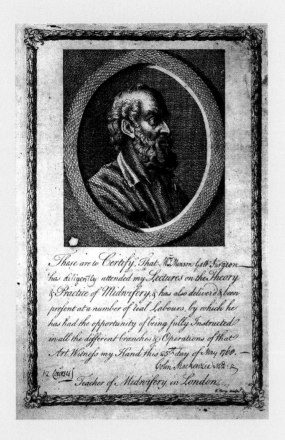

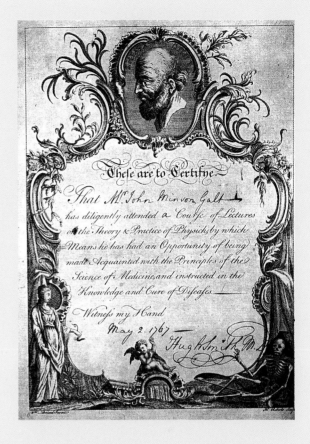

Dr. Galt was appointed a visiting physician to the Public Hospital after Dr. John de Sequeyra died in 1795 and to the hospital's court of directors in 1799. The Galt family maintained a long medical association with the hospital. John Minson's brother, James, had been appointed keeper twenty-three years earlier; John's son, Alexander, also a visiting physician, worked there for some years with his father. John Minson Galt II, Alexander's son, became superintendent of the hospital in 1841 and held the post until his untimely death in 1862.

John Minson Galt died at the age of sixty-four on June 12, 1808, after practicing medicine for forty years. His obituary noted that Galt enjoyed "a reputation and success of very uncommon distinction."[56]

Left: "These are to Certify That Mr. J. Minson Galt Surgeon has diligently attended my Lectures on the Theory & Practice of Midwifery & has also deliver'd & been present at a number of real Labours, by which he has had the opportunity of being fully Instructed in all the different branches & Operations of that Art, Witness my Hand this 25th day of May 1768. Colin Mackenzie M.D. 12 Courses Teacher of Midwifery in London."

Right: "These are to Certifye That Mr John Minson Galt has diligently attended a Course of Lectures on the Theory & Practice of Physick, by which Means he has had an Opportunity of being made Acquainted with the Principles of the Science of Medicine and instructed in the Knowledge and Cure of Diseases. Witness my Hand May 2, 1767 Hugh Smith M.D."

not discovered until the 1840s, a surgeon needed to complete his procedures quickly to lessen the patient's pain and minimize blood loss and shock. Infection was prevalent after surgery. Knowledge of antiseptic measures would not be developed until the second half of the nineteenth century.

Midwifery

"Midwifery, in the largest sense of the word, implies the art of assisting a child-bearing woman, before, in the time of, and after her labour is over."[57] Traditionally, midwives assumed the responsibility for most deliveries.

Catherine Blaikley, a well-known Williamsburg midwife, had a long and distinguished career. An obituary in October 1771 described the widow Blaikley as "an eminent Midwife" who had "brought upwards of three Thousand Children into the World."[58] Mary Rose, the wife of a faculty member at William and Mary, advertised in the local newspaper. Mary Roberts, a free mulatto midwife, lived near Carter's Grove plantation.[59] One or more slave women may also have practiced midwifery at Carter's Grove.[60] Unfortunately, none of them left a diary.

It was important for a midwife to have a basic understanding of anatomy, know how to deliver the placenta, and be able to recognize potential problems. Doctors thought that midwives did not need in-depth training in handling complications or obstetrical tools. If a serious condition developed, a midwife was expected to ask a doctor for assistance.

Experience was generally gained by attending deliveries and, on occasion, dissections. Books written specifically for midwives such as John Culpepper's *A Directory for Midwives*, which was advertised in the *Virginia Gazette*, were available. While some midwives learned from female practitioners, others studied with doctors.

Mary Rose advertised that she had completed her training, about which nothing is known, under Doctors Pasteur and Galt:

Having studied and practised MIDWIFERY for some Time past, with Success, under the Direction, and with the Approbation, of Doctors Pasteur and Galt, flatters herself she will meet with Encouragement, as Nothing will be spared to complete her in the Knowledge of an Art so eminently necessary to the Good of Mankind. Ladies, and others, are therefore desired to take Notice that they will be waited upon on the shortest Warning, by their humble Servant.[61]

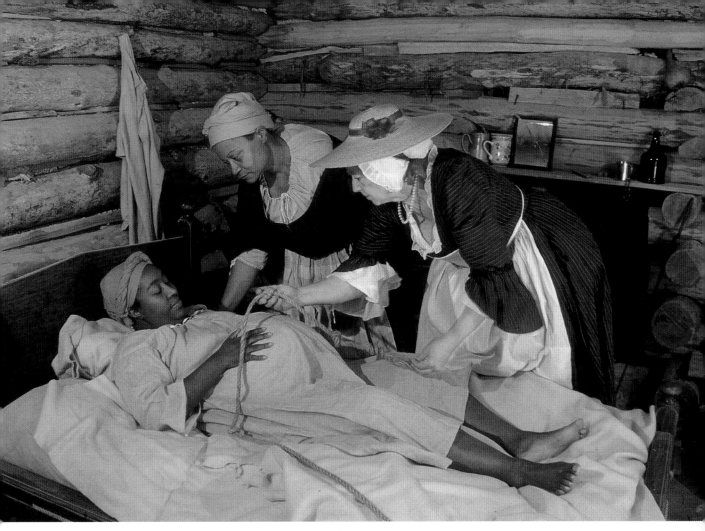

Pregnant slaves received care from midwives, their owners, and, on occasion, a man-midwife. The status of the mother determined whether the child was a slave or free.

By the 1760s, a change in the preference for birth attendants was becoming evident. Upper-class women in large cities such as Philadelphia, New York, Boston, and London were choosing male doctors to attend their normal deliveries. Some patients believed that a doctor's specialized training enabled him to provide a safer delivery. Doctors were discovering that most births were normal, and the fees for their midwifery services provided another source of income.

Williamsburg had its share of man-midwives too. In addition to John Galt, George Gilmer, Jr., Andrew Anderson, and Peter Hay advertised midwifery services. Although Dr. Alexander Middleton owned obstetrical instruments, it is not clear if he actually practiced as a man-midwife.

In the colonies, formal training in midwifery was available at King's College in New York when it opened in 1767. Dr. William Shippen, Jr. (1736–1808), advertised classes in 1763 and 1765 in Philadelphia. During this time, London doctors had a widespread reputation for teaching midwifery. While John Galt was in London, he studied with Colin Mackenzie. Mackenzie (d. 1775) had trained with Dr. William Smellie (1697–1763), a leader in midwifery education. Insight into the content of Mackenzie's lectures survives in letters of his American pupil, Samuel Bard:

His Method was first to give a History of Midwifry, then the Description of the Pelvis, and Parts of Generation, and . . . some hints on Conception; he then procedes to an account of the Gravid [pregnant] Uterus and the Disorders of Women During pregnancy; after Discribes the true signs of labour and the requisites to a natural one, after

After Dr. Galt finished his training in midwifery, surgery, and medicine in London, he returned to Williamsburg and placed this advertisement in the *Virginia Gazette*.

THE subscriber, who is just arrived from LONDON, purposes settling in WILLIAMSBURG, where he intends practising as a SURGEON, APOTHECARY, and MAN-MIDWIFE; and hopes, from the application he has made in these branches, to be able to give satisfaction. Those who will please to favour him with their employ may depend upon the strictest attendance. JOHN MINSON GALT.

To be SOLD, *on* Wednesday *the* 22d *of this instant* February,

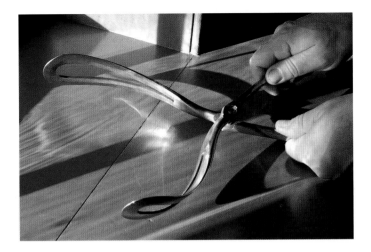

Professional texts recommended the use of obstetric forceps only for emergencies, including hemorrhaging and convulsions.

this he gives a practical touching Lecture, and another upon the Various Instruments, of which he shows a great Collection; points out the different improvements, & mentions their Inventors, he intirely Discards many from practice, and recommends but few, and those to be used with the greatest Caution; only in Cases of Necessity—he next procedes to the Delivery of Both natural and preternatural Cases upon Machinery, then gives Directions for the management of the Patient in Labour, & During the Month, Discribes the Dissorders Incident to them at this time, and the Method of Cure, and Concludes his Course with the Dissorders Insident to the Infant, & some Directions, with regard to the choice of a Nurse.[62]

"Touching" involved inserting one or two fingers into the birth canal to determine how far labor had progressed, what part of the infant presented, and if the membranes had broken. Practitioners learned the procedure by practicing with machines or mannequins made of leather that served as models of the pelvic region. Touching was an important aspect of training because it enabled the man-midwife to follow the progress of the delivery. Students also learned to turn the baby and deliver it by the feet, to use forceps, and, in extremely difficult cases, how to save the mother's life by dismembering the fetus. Aspiring man-midwives were informed about cesarean sections, delivering twins, hemorrhaging, and difficult presentations.

Dr. Mackenzie saw to it that his students received clinical experience. The patients were often indigent women who were willing to have their deliveries attended by a teacher and students in exchange for free medical care. Pupils received certificates at the conclusion of the training.

Of the several man-midwives in Williamsburg, only Dr. Galt's records have survived. Samples from his daybook include sketchy details such as "Examing & advice woman in Lab.," "Midwifry," "attendce midwifery Visit Woman," "Visit in the night & delivery Placenta Nelly."[63] Nelly's case is one of the rare instances when a specific complication was mentioned.

While early eighteenth-century practitioners felt it was necessary to remove the placenta immediately after delivery, by the late 1760s, most practitioners recommended allowing the placenta time to detach itself before trying to remove it manually. Dr. Mackenzie preferred to wait for about an hour unless the condition was serious and the patient started hemorrhaging. Since Galt did not make a habit of recording case notes in his daybook, there is no way to tell if he followed his teacher's advice or removed the placenta as quickly as possible.

Other situations that practitioners found especially challenging included cases of childbed fever, patients who wanted to terminate a pregnancy, and ectopic (non-uterine) pregnancies. It is important to remember that, by eighteenth-century standards, most births were considered normal and mothers generally survived deliveries.

Summary

Surviving records provide a window on the practice of medicine in a colonial town. Williamsburg daybooks tell of house calls in the middle of the night to prescribe medications, dispense advice, or occasionally to perform surgery. *Virginia Gazette*s reported the arrival of drugs and sundries for sale, the concern over a smallpox epidemic, and the start of a new medical practice or partnership. Newspapers printed obituaries of practitioners and announced sales of their estates. Evidence of training through apprenticeships and attendance at English hospitals and European universities survives in contracts, newspaper advertisements, and certificates. Inventories list surgical tools, drugs, and pharmaceutical equipment. Medical textbooks by leading authors contain the signatures of their local owners.

Other records chronicle the attempts to regulate the practice of medicine and doctors' fees in Virginia. Professional licensing was for-

PETER HAY (1712?–1766)

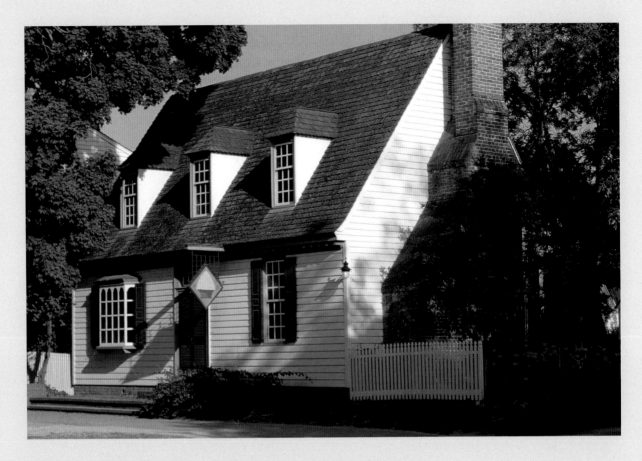

From 1744 until his death, Dr. Peter Hay[64] operated a shop in Williamsburg next to the Market Square. While his medical training is not known, obituaries in the *Virginia* and *Maryland Gazette*s described him as one of the city's "most eminent physicians"[65] and noted that he had "for many Years practised Midwifery with great Success."[66] In addition to his home and shop in Williamsburg, Dr. Hay owned a plantation in neighboring King William County where he sold several head of cattle, some horses, and more than twenty slaves at auction in 1745.[67]

Although Dr. Hay's apothecary shop on Duke of Gloucester Street burned to the ground in 1756, he continued to practice medicine. In 1766, Hay died in his home at the age of fifty-four. The inventory of his goods included several more slaves, a fine chariot, household furniture, and a "choice library of books"[68] that were auctioned off after his death. Like many other widows of the time, Mrs. Hay turned their home into a lodging house.

Dr. Peter Hay's shop has been reconstructed on Duke of Gloucester Street.

mally discussed and then rejected in the 1770s. Thomas Jefferson's proposal to establish a medical school at William and Mary was unsuccessful. However, the proposal to build a "lunatic asylum" resulted in the opening of the first publicly funded mental hospital in the colonies.

Archeological research has unearthed medical paraphernalia used by Williamsburg apothecaries and land records confirm the locations of their shops, thereby enabling the reconstruction of some sites. Descendants of several colonial practitioners and legislators have given researchers access to their ancestors' books and personal papers.

What do these newspaper accounts, pottery fragments, daybooks, and inventories mean to us today? Individually, they represent artifacts from our past. Collectively, they tell the story of an era in which people were searching for new ways to treat the timeless problems of the human condition and were creating new medical theories based on the latest scientific discoveries.

Notes

1 James Parker to Charles Steuart, Dec. 1770, manuscript 5040, microfilm reel 68.9, John D. Rockefeller, Jr. Library, Colonial Williamsburg Foundation.

2 Dr. de Sequeyra's "Account of Virginia Diseases, 1745–1781," in Harold B. Gill, Jr., *The Apothecary in Colonial Virginia* (Williamsburg, Va., 1972), p. 110.

3 Parker to Steuart, Dec. 1770.

4 Daybook of John Minson Galt, Nov. 26, 1792, Galt Family Papers, MS books, 1767–1796, microfilm reel 1131.16, Rockefeller Lib.

5 Account book of John Minson Galt, ca. 1770–1775, pp. 10, 12, 14, 58, 3, 25, Galt Family Papers, microfilm reel 1079, Rockefeller Lib.

6 *Virginia Gazette* (Williamsburg) (Purdie & Dixon), Feb. 25, 1773.

7 *Ibid.*, May 20, 1773.

8 *Ibid.*, May 13, 1773.

9 *Va. Gaz.* (Williamsburg) (Dixon & Hunter), June 6, 1777.

10 Apprentice indenture of Frederick Bryan to Dr. John Minson Galt, Nov. 16, 1778, York County, Va., Records, Deed Book VI, 1777–1791, p. 15, in Gill, *Apothecary*, p. 61.

11 George Gilmer to Hill and Lamer, Nov. 3, 1755, *ibid.*, p. 55.

12 William Langhorne, Address to the Virginia Legislature Concerning the Requirement of Licensing for those Practicing Medicine, 1772–1775, p. 4, courtesy, W. T. Langhorne.

13 His date of birth must have been ca. 1717 since McKenzie is assumed to have been 21 when he married in 1738. His will, dated Feb. 8, 1755, is recorded in the York Co. Recs., Will Book XX, p. 352. This information was collected in the York County Master Biographical File under Grants RS-00033-80-1604 and RO-20869-85 from the National Endowment for the Humanities to the Department of Historical Research, CWF.

14 Hermann Boerhaave, *Dr. Boerhaave's Academical Lectures on the Theory of Physic*, I (London, 1742), pp. 2–3.

15 William Cullen, *A Synopsis of Methodical Nosology*, trans. Henry Wilkins from the 4th ed. (Philadelphia, 1793), p. iii.

16 R. Brookes, *The General Practice of Physic*, I, 3rd ed. (London, 1758), p. 1.

17 *Ibid.*, p. 2.

18 *Ibid.*

19 *Ibid.*, pp. 4–5.

20 William Cullen, *First Lines of the Practice of Physic*, I, 2nd ed. (Philadelphia, 1781), p. 229.

21 Brookes, *General Practice of Physic*, p. 2.

22 *Ibid.*, p. 3.

23 Gill, *Apothecary*, pp. 96–115. "Intermittent" refers to any type of fever that comes and goes at regular intervals.

24 *Ibid.*

25 York Co. Recs., Deed Book VIII, 1769–1777, pp. 236–238, CWF. The site where Dr. de Sequeyra lived is today occupied by Shields Tavern.

26 *Virginia Gazette and General Advertiser* (Richmond) (Davis), Mar. 18, 1795.

27 Peter Shaw, *A New Practice of Physic*, 3rd ed. (London, 1730), p. iv.

28 George Cheyne, *An Essay on Regimen* (London, 1740), p. iv.

29 *Ibid.*, p. lx.

30 Brookes, *General Practice of Physic*, p. 47.

31 William Pasteur's birth date is assumed to have been by ca. 1737 because he witnessed a deed in 1753 and a person had to be at least 16 in order to do so. York Co. Master Biog. File, CWF.

32 Wyndham B. Blanton, *Medicine in Virginia in the Eighteenth Century* (Richmond, Va., 1931), p. 322.

33 William Stith Pasteur's birth record is listed in the Bruton Parish Records. Dr. Pasteur's will indicates that he died "childless." York Co. Master Biog. File, CWF.

34 *Va. Gaz.* (Purdie & Dixon), Apr. 15, 1775.

35 *Va. Gaz.* (Williamsburg) (Rind), Sept. 21, 1769.

36 J. Worth Estes, *Dictionary of Protopharmacology* (Canton, Mass., 1990), p. 51.

37 *Ibid.*, pp. 98, 99.

38 *Every Man his own Doctor: or, The Poor Planter's Physician*, 3rd ed. (Williamsburg, Va., 1736), pp. 70-71.

39 The birth date of George Gilmer, Sr., has not definitely been established. The *William and Mary* Quarterly, 1st Ser., XV (1906–1907), p. 225, stated that Gilmer was born in 1700 in Edinburgh but gave no source. His birth date was listed as "by 1711" in the York Co. Recs., Wills, but this is based on his first recorded marriage in Williamsburg in 1732. Gilmer had to be at least 21 before he could marry legally in Virginia. The date of his marriage to Mary Peachy Walker would therefore place his birth date in 1711 or earlier.

40 *WMQ*, 1st Ser., XV (1906–1907), p. 225. Gilmer may have married in London before emigrating to Williamsburg.

41 Gilmer Family Bible, York Co. Recs., Wills.

42 R. Butler, *An Essay Concerning Blood-Letting* (London, 1734), p. 30.

43 John Quincy, *Pharmacopeia Officinalis & Extemporaneous, Or, A Complete English Dispensatory*, 5th ed. (London, 1724), p. 234.

44 Hugh Smith, *Essays Physiological and Practical, on the Nature and Circulation of the Blood* (London, 1761), p. 61.

45 William Buchan, *Domestic Medicine; or, The Family Physician*, 2nd American ed. (Philadelphia, 1774), reprint (New York, 1993), p. 421.

46 *Va. Gaz.* (Purdie & Dixon), Jan. 2, 1772.

47 Pierre Fauchard, *The Surgeon Dentist; or, Treatise on the Teeth*, 2nd ed. (Paris, 1746), reprint (Pound Ridge, N. J., 1946), p. 28.

48 *Va. Gaz.* (Purdie & Dixon), Oct. 10, 1771.

49 *Va. Gaz.* (Williamsburg) (Purdie), Apr. 21, 1775.

50 Claim of Alexander Middleton, Mar. 25, 1784, Loyalist Claims, 1776–1789, P.R.O./A.O., 13-31.

51 *Va. Gaz.* (Purdie & Dixon), Jan. 13, 1774.

52 *Ibid.*, Dec. 13, 1770.

53 *Va. Gaz. and Gen. Adv.* (Davis), June 3, 1773.

54 Writings of Sally Galt, pp. 3, 4, Galt Family Papers, microfilm reel 1131.13, Rockefeller Lib.

55 *Va. Gaz.* (Purdie & Dixon), Sept. 21, 1769.

56 *Va. Gaz. and Gen. Adv.* (Davis), June 24, 1808.

57 John Memis, *The Midwife's Pocket-Companion: Or a Practical Treatise of Midwifery* (London, 1765), n.p.

58 *Va. Gaz.* (Purdie & Dixon), Oct. 24, 1771.

59 Lorena S. Walsh, *From Calabar to Carter's Grove: The History of a Virginia Slave Community* (Charlottesville, Va., 1997), p. 175.

60 *Ibid.*

61 *Va. Gaz.* (Purdie & Dixon), Jan. 9, 1772. The reference to "others" has been interpreted by some to mean that Mary Rose also delivered slave women.

62 Jane B. Donegan, *Women & Men Midwives: Medicine, Morality, and Misogyny in Early America* (Westport, Conn., 1978), p. 103.

63 Galt Daybook, Feb. 6, 22, Mar. 19, 30, 1784, microfilm reel 1131.16, Rockefeller Lib. Nelly is believed to have been a slave who was owned by William Holt.

64 In 1752, Peter Hay testified in the court case of Lewis and Frances Burrel *vs.* Phillip and Elizabeth Smith. The record stated that Hay was "40 years of age," making his birth year 1712. British Museum MS. Add. MS 36, 218, pp. 138-143, microfilm reel 284, York Co. Recs., CWF.

65 *Va. Gaz.* (Purdie & Dixon), Nov. 27, 1766.

66 *Ibid.* (Rind), Nov. 27, 1766.

67 *Ibid.* (Parks), Nov. 21, 1745.

68 *Ibid.* (Purdie & Dixon), Feb. 26, 1767.

Further Reading

David L. Cowen and William H. Helfand. *Pharmacy: An Illustrated History*. New York: Harry N. Abrams, Inc., 1990.

Andrew Cunningham and Roger French, eds. *The Medical Enlightenment of the Eighteenth Century*. Cambridge: Cambridge University Press, 1990.

Donald R. Hopkins. *Princes and Peasants: Smallpox in History*. Chicago: University of Chicago Press, 1983.

Lester S. King. *The Medical World of the Eighteenth Century*. Chicago: University of Chicago Press, 1958.

Judith Walzer Leavitt. *Brought to Bed: Childbearing In America, 1750 to 1950*. New York: Oxford University Press, 1986.

Malvin E. Ring. *Dentistry: An Illustrated History*. New York: Harry N. Abrams, Inc., 1985.

Lisa M. Rosner. *Medical Education in the Age of Improvement: Edinburgh Students and Apprentices 1760–1826*. Edinburgh: Edinburgh University Press, 1991.

Ira M. Rutkow. *Surgery: An Illustrated History*. St. Louis: Mosby-Year Book, Inc., 1993.

Shomer S. Zwelling. *Quest for a Cure: The Public Hospital in Williamsburg, Virginia, 1773–1885*. Williamsburg, Va.: Colonial Williamsburg Foundation, 1985.